RINGWORM

How to Identify Ringworm, Treat It, and Stay Dermatologically Strong: The Ringworm Handbook

CHAD BRUNO

Table of Contents

Introductory

The fungus that causes ringworm can infect the skin, the hair, or the nails. The disease is really caused by a number of different fungus despite its worm-like moniker. Since the raised, red rash that typically accompanies ringworm might be misinterpreted as either a ring or a worm, the term "ringworm" was coined to describe this condition.

• Ringworm can infect people and animals and is very contagious. Common symptoms include itchiness, redness, and scaling, making the affected region quite unpleasant. Ringworm, also known as tinea capitis, tinea corporis, tinea pedis, or athlete's foot, and tinea cruris, or jock itch, can manifest on several body parts. The nails (tinea unguium) may also be affected.

Antifungal drugs are commonly used to treat ringworm, either topically or orally depending on the severity of the illness. If you feel you have ringworm and want to get rid of it without spreading it to others, you should consult a doctor to get a proper diagnosis and treatment plan.

CHAPTER ONE
Intro to Ringworm

Contrary to popular belief, fungi, not worms, are responsible for ringworm. The following is a brief primer on ringworm:

• ringworm is a fungal infection that can manifest itself in a number of ways (including but not limited to the skin, hair, and nails). The fungi responsible for ringworm are typically of the dermatophyte group.

Named for the distinctive rash it causes, "ringworm" describes the outward manifestation of this skin infection. It can cause a rash that looks like a ring or a worm: red, elevated, and circular on the outside with clear or normal skin in the middle. This circular look is not always evident, yet the moniker "ringworm" persists.

• It's contagious people can catch it from each other or from animals, and it can spread quickly. Towels, combs, and clothing can all harbor the virus and spread it to others.

Different varieties of ringworm result from the fact that it can manifest in different places on the body.

Tinea corporis is a bodily condition.

• Hair and scalp infection known as tinea capitis.

Commonly known as "athlete's foot," o Tinea Pedis attacks the feet.

• Tinea Cruris: Known as jock itch, it affects the groin area.

Involvement of the nails; Tinea Unguium.

• Symptoms Itching, redness, and scaling are typical reactions to ringworm. It's not pleasant and may even result in painful blisters or pus-filled sores.

Antifungal medicines are the standard approach to treating ringworm. Depending on the severity and location of the illness, the therapy may be topical (given to the skin) or systemic (administered orally). Mild infections usually respond well to over-the-counter antifungal treatments, while more serious infections may require prescription drugs.

- **Hygiene and Prevention:** Keeping the affected region clean and dry, as well as practicing proper personal hygiene, will help prevent the spread of ringworm and other fungal infections. In addition to timely treatment and isolation, rapid containment is essential.

• Seek the Advice of a Medical Expert: Seek professional medical help for a confirmed diagnosis and effective treatment of ringworm. The diagnosis of ringworm should be confirmed by a medical practitioner so that they can provide the most effective treatment.

Despite its prevalence, ringworm is a manageable fungal condition that can be cured with the right treatment.

Most Typical Signs

Depending on the type and location of the infection, the symptoms of ringworm can change. Common symptoms of several forms of ringworm include:

1. Tinea corporis, often known as ringworm of the body, is characterized by the appearance of a red, circular or oval rash.

• Skin irritation and itch.

• A depression in the middle, giving the impression of a ring.

Scaling, edging up.

• Pustules and blisters are a possibility.

2. Tinea Capitis (Scalp Ringworm): Patches of itchy, scaly, or irritated scalp.

• Your hair could dry out and break easily.

• Patches of baldness or general hair loss in the area.

• Sometimes, there are enlarged lymph nodes.

3. Athlete's foot, also known as tinea pedis, is characterized by: o stinging and burning between the

toes, most noticeably the fourth and fifth.

• Dry skin that flakes, peels, and cracks on the foot.

• Sole inflammation and blistering.

The feet smell bad.

Tinea cruris, often known as jock itch, is a rash that typically appears in the groin and inner thigh and is itchy, red, and round.

• Rash may extend down the inner thighs.

• The rash may have elevated margins and a central clearing at times.

5. Nail ringworm (Tinea unguium):

Nails (often toenails) thicken, change color, and become brittle.

Nail discoloration; white or yellow patches.

- Fraying or sharp corners.

- Nail deformation.

Seeing a doctor for a diagnosis and treatment is recommended because ringworm symptoms might be similar to those of other skin disorders. To effectively manage and eradicate ringworm, early diagnosis and adequate treatment are crucial. It's also crucial to take precautions against spreading ringworm because of its contagious nature.

CHAPTER TWO
Care and Preventative Measures

Different types of ringworm infections require different approaches to treatment and prevention. General recommendations for dealing with and avoiding ringworm are as follows:

Treatment:

Antifungal drugs are the first line of defense against ringworm. The nature and severity of an illness will determine whether a topical (applied to the skin) or systemic (given orally) therapy is more appropriate.

OTC antifungal creams, lotions, and ointments such clotrimazole, terbinafine, and miconazole may be useful for mild instances. Put these on the affected region and leave them there for as long as instructed.

Topical medicines or systemic antifungal agents of prescription strength may be necessary for more severe or widespread infections. The right course of treatment will be decided by your doctor.

Oral antifungal drugs like griseofulvin, terbinafine, or itraconazole may be administered in some circumstances, particularly for infections of the scalp (tinea capitis) or severe cases of ringworm. Always listen to your doctor's advice on dosage and length of treatment.

Keep the area clean and dry to cut off the fungus's food source, and you'll be well on your way to eradicating the problem. It needs to be washed and dried daily with care. Don't lend or borrow your clothes, combs, or towels to others.

• **Isolation:** If you or your pet have ringworm, it's best to limit your interactions with other people and animals until treatment has begun and the infection is no longer contagious.

Prevention:

First, always wash your hands with soap and water after coming into contact with animals, utilizing shared spaces, or anything else that could spread the fungus.

Fungi grow in warm, damp environments, so it's important to keep your skin dry. Preventing ringworm requires keeping the skin dry, especially in sweaty regions. If you need to, you can use antifungal powders.

Don't share towels, clothes, or personal grooming products with someone who has ringworm.

Those with ringworm should wash and disinfect their clothes, blankets, and towels frequently. Wash your clothes in hot water using a high-quality detergent. Personal objects such as hairbrushes and combs should be sterilized.

• Always use clean, dry socks and shoes with good ventilation to prevent athlete's foot. Do not go shoeless in public places like showers or pools.

Check and treat your pets for ringworm on a regular basis, especially cats and dogs. See a vet immediately if you suspect your pet has an infection.

Seventh, keep your distance from animals that may be contaminated, and remember to wash your hands and any other exposed skin after coming into contact with an animal.

Keep in mind that managing and stopping the spread of ringworm requires quick diagnosis and treatment. If you suspect you have ringworm or see signs in your pet, speak with a healthcare specialist or veterinarian for guidance.

Outside the Body

Because ringworm infections can spread beyond the skin and damage other organs, it's crucial to note that the term "ringworm" is often used interchangeably with other medical names for describing specific fungal illnesses. Extracutaneous manifestations of ringworm include the following:

• Form of ringworm infection that manifests on the scalp and hair is called tinea capitis. There may be hair loss, itchy, scaly, or inflammatory spots on the scalp, and even lymph node swelling. Ringworm of the scalp most commonly affects kids, but it can happen to anyone.

• Nail fungus known as tinea unguium can affect either the

toenails or, less frequently, the fingernails. Nails that are infected may thicken, change color, become brittle, or show signs of infection such as white or yellow streaks. It may be necessary to take oral antifungal medicine to effectively treat a fungal infection of the nails.

• **Tinea Corporis (Body Ringworm):** this condition typically manifests as a localized skin infection, but in those with compromised immune systems, it can spread to other areas of the body.

• **Systemic fungal infections:** Some kinds of ringworm and other fungal diseases can spread throughout the body and into the bloodstream. This is particularly common in persons with impaired immune systems, such as those with HIV/AIDS, cancer, or organ transplant recipients.

• **Kerion:** This is a painful, swelling, and swampy mass on the scalp caused by a severe case of tinea capitis (scalp ringworm). It can cause scarring if left untreated and requires prompt treatment with oral antifungal drugs.

If you think you have a fungal infection deeper than the skin, you should see a doctor right once since you may need specialized care. Many fungal infections may be diagnosed by a doctor, who can then advise on the best course of treatment, which may include oral antifungal drugs and the correction of any underlying health problems that may be causing or aggravating the illness.

The likelihood of developing a life-threatening or systemic fungal infection is diminished when proper hygiene is practiced, measures are taken to limit the spread of infection, and underlying health issues are addressed. Seek medical attention immediately if you or a loved one exhibits symptoms that may point to these diseases.

Conclusion

As a fungal infection, ringworm can manifest itself on the skin, hair, and nails of both humans and animals. The disease is actually caused by a number of different fungi, despite its misleading name. The rash often takes the form of a ring or circle, but can take on other shapes or sizes depending on the cause and severity of the infection.

Depending on the severity of the illness, antifungal medicines may be used topically or taken orally to treat ringworm. Early diagnosis and adequate treatment are critical to manage and eliminate ringworm successfully.

Good hygiene, not sharing towels or bedding, keeping the infected region clean and dry, and getting treatment quickly can all help stop the spread of ringworm.

In people with compromised immune systems, ringworm can spread to the scalp and nails and potentially trigger systemic fungal illnesses. These illnesses call for the expertise of trained medical professionals.

For proper diagnosis and treatment of ringworm or a related fungal infection, it is recommended that you see a doctor or veterinarian (in the case of dogs). Ringworm is a common fungal infection that can be avoided with proper cleanliness and preventative measures.

THE END